LET'S WORK IT OUT

A PROBLEM-SOLVING JOURNAL

DR. LILA SWELL

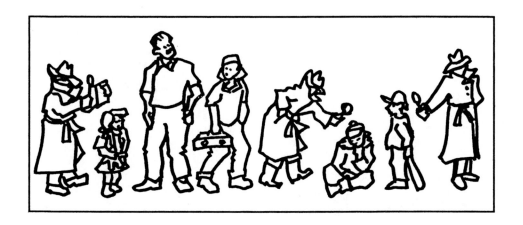

ILLUSTRATED BY MARSHA LIPSITZ

Book Design by Ronnie Tuft

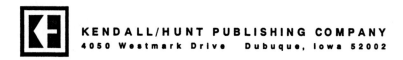

KENDALL/HUNT PUBLISHING COMPANY
4050 Westmark Drive   Dubuque, Iowa 52002

Cover photo courtesy of Barry Frank

Table of Contents

Introduction to Students

The purpose of this Journal is to help you to become a better "Problem Solver" and to develop positive values.

There are a series of exercises to help you learn how to understand and communicate your feelings and thoughts in positive ways.

Problem-solving is a two-way street. You will learn to become more sensitive to other people's feelings and to figure out the underlying thoughts and feelings which prompts their behavior.

Self-discipline is also part of Problem-Solving, so you will learn how to control your own thoughts and feelings and how to channel them into positive action. You will learn to act thoughtfully, not impulsively. The solution to a problem is rarely a simple, one-step process because most problems are more complicated than they appear. You will learn how to identify the *real*, as opposed to the *superficial*, problem.

In addition, you will be learning about "values" because your values affect the choice of solutions to a problem that you may make. There are exercises in this Journal which are designed to help you to identify your own personal set of values, your "value system". You will be exposed to many new positive values which you may wish to integrate into your present set of values.

With your new, improved Problem-Solving skills, you can make decisions which will result in a better world for you and your generation, as well as for future generations.

Bill of Rights

I Have The Right To Say "No".

I Have The Right To Ask For Help.

*I Have The Right To Ask Others To
Correct Mistakes That Effect Me.*

I Have The Right To Make Mistakes.

I Have The Right To Make Choices.

*I Have The Right To My Own Tastes,
Opinions, Attitudes And Beliefs.*

*I Have The Right To Express My
Feelings To Others In Positive Ways.*

*I Have The Right To Protect Myself
From Verbal And Physical Abuse.*

*I Have The Right To Make My Feelings
And Needs Known.*

The above is a list of your rights. You must be aware of your rights before you can begin to solve your problems.

face your feelings

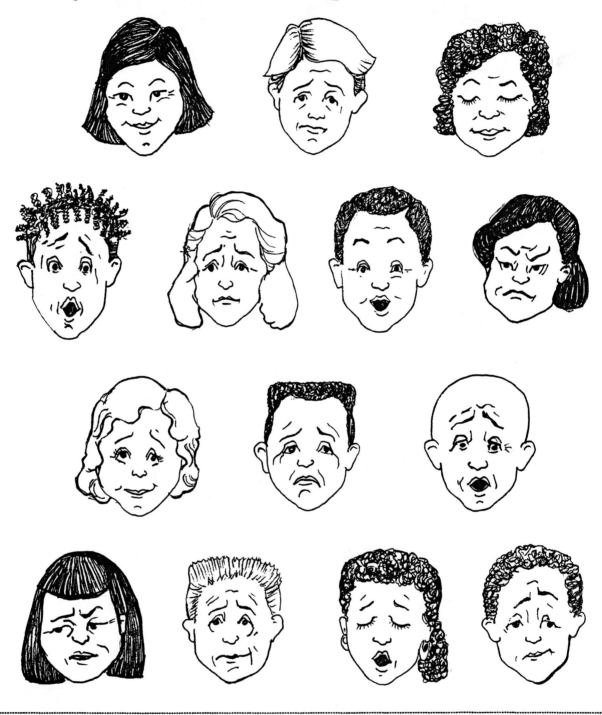

Happy	*Confident*	*Calm*	*Jealous*	*Joyful*	*Frustrated*
Sad	*Frightened*	*Angry*	*Rejected*	*Excited*	*Eager*
Proud	*Surprised*	*Helpless*	*Hopeful*	*Bored*	*Love Struc*
Confused	*Guilty*	*Peaceful*	*Worried*	*Sorry*	*Glad*

face your feelings

Look at the "Feeling Faces" and the "Feeling List" on the opposite page. What do you think each face is ~~ing?~~ Write your interpretation below each face.
On this page, choose the feeling that you might have in the following situations:

I won a prize. I feel -

The teacher pays more attention to the other students. I feel -

I got 100% on the spelling test. I feel -

The water is too deep and I'm not a good swimmer. I feel -

My Grandfather drinks too much. I feel -

I forgot to get my best friend a birthday present. I feel -

My bike was broken and I fixed it myself. I feel -

. I live with a foster family. I feel -

. My family and I don't fight as much as we used to. I feel -

. My friend was mugged. I feel -

describe your feelings

Write about something that has happened recently that caused you to have one or more of the feelings from the "Feeling List".

Describe what happened:

. . . .

. . . .

. . . .

. . . .

. . . .

. . . .

Describe how it made you feel:

. . . .

. . . .

. . . .

. . . .

. . . .

TURN IT AROUND.
Sometimes a "negative" feeling can be used for a "positive" action which can turn a "negative" feeling into a "positive" feeling.
Example:

> "I was jealous of the attention given the players on our team. It made me practice harder to prove I could make the team. The next time, at the try-outs, I played so well that I made the team."

Can you "turn around" any of the above experiences that left you with "negative" feelings?

. . . .

. . . .

Let's Work It

draw your feelings

In the face below, draw yourself showing the feelings you wrote about. Add all the details that make it look like you. Refer to the "Feeling Faces" on page 6.

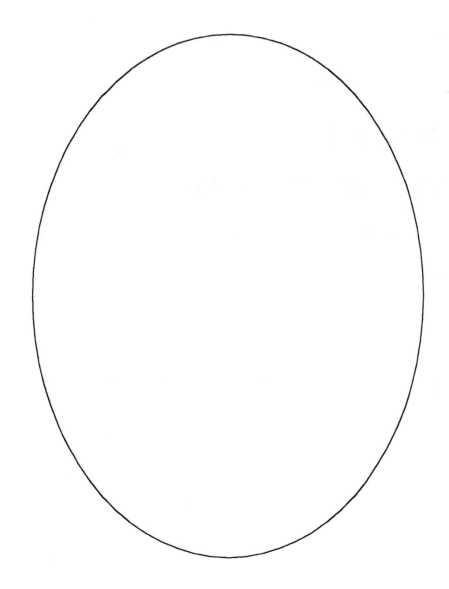

PEP TALK. . . . .
ways to change your thinking

Apply the following steps in the next set of exercises. This will help you to examine your thoughts and turn negative thoughts into positive ones.

1. Recognize the thoughts that upset you.

2. Set aside time to think about what's bothering you.

3. Write down your negative thoughts--the words you say to yourself.

4. Do not judge yourself as a "bad" person.

5. STOP the negative thoughts.

6. Substitute positive thoughts for negative thoughts.

7. Live NOW, in the present, not in the past or in the future.

8. Make positive statements to yourself.

Before moving on to the exercises, read the examples below which describe POSITIVE and NEGATIVE Self Talk. They will help you to see the difference between the two more clearly.

Examples of positive and negative Self Talk:

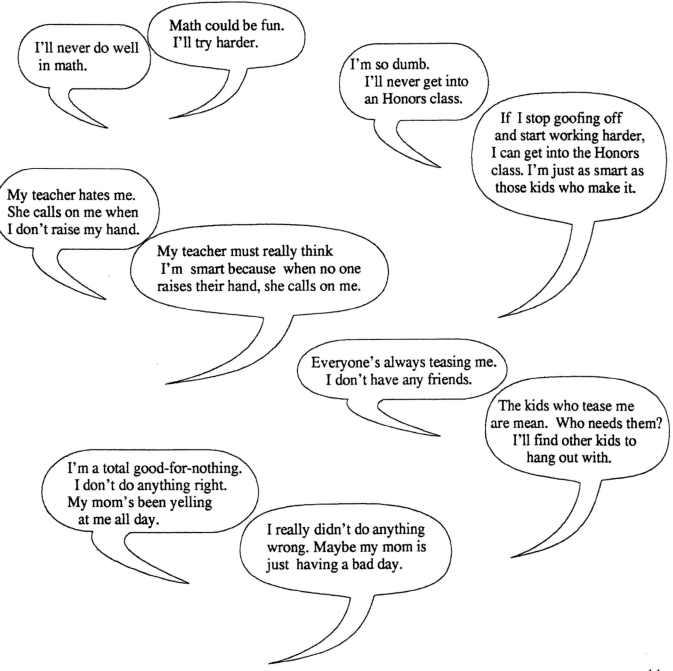

Pep Talk. . . . .

Think of an experience that made you feel badly. In the space below write about your experience and feelings, and what you said to yourself.

Experience:

....

....

....

....

....

Feelings:

....

....

....

....

Negative Self Talk:

....

....

....

....

In the blank below, write down what you could say to yourself to make you feel better.

Positive Self Talk:

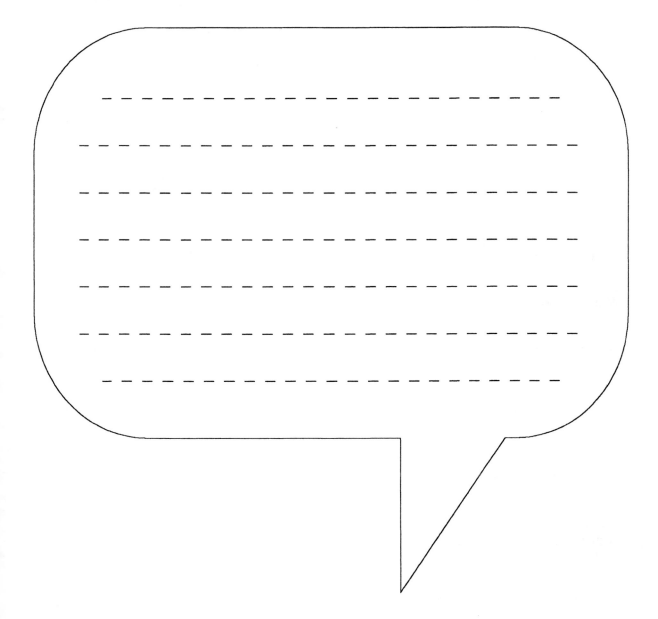

The following is a list of "You and I Messages". Read the messages and the rules at the bottom of the page before doing the exercise on the opposite page.

"YOU"   ## "I"

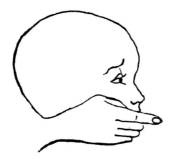   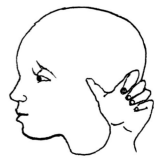

"You don't take care of yourself."   "I'm concerned about you."

"You're confusing me."   "I don't understand what you want."

"You're not working hard enough."   "I'm worried that things won't get finished on time."

"You should be ashamed of the way you are behaving."   "I'm embarrassed by your behavior."

"You never say 'Thank you'."   I feel unappreciated."

"You think I'm stupid."   "I don't know if I'm capable of doing what you want."

"You are giving me too much homework."   "I'm feeling overwhelmed and I don't know if I'll be able to finish the assignment."

"You" messages are used to express commands, criticism, blame, and punishment

But "You" messages can also express: hidden anger, fault finding, or not being able to accept responsibility

---

"I" messages express:

+ true and honest feelings
+ non-judgemental concern
+ readiness to be helpful
+ understanding another's feelings

Pretend that someone is saying these things to you. Write an "I" message expressing the feeling inside the blank bubble.

"YOU"   "I"

MPLE:

You are paying more attention to my brother than to me.

I'm feeling neglected and not cared for.

You make the tests too hard.

You don't explain things clearly.

You never call me.

You eat too much candy.

You keep me waiting. You're never on time!

Listening with your HEART

A simple statement may sometimes reveal more than one feeling. Match the statements that are in the SOMEONE SAYS column with as many feelings in the second column that you think reveal that person's deepest feelings.

Draw lines that connect the statements to the underlying feelings.

SOMEONE SAYS . . .

"I have too much
homework to do."

"I have to do what my friends
tell me to do."

"I hate you!"

"My sister always gets
nicer presents than I do."

"It's a 'man's' world".

"I tried so hard in math,
but I still failed".

"If I don't do drugs or steal,
my friends will call me 'chicken'."

"My mother is hardly
ever at home."

"The teacher never calls on me
to answer questions."

"She likes him better
than she likes me."

"I didn't mean to hurt him
when I pushed him."

. . . FEELINGS

remorseful

intimidated

lonely

jealous

helpless

angry

overlooked

fear of losing "status"

overwhelmed

unloved

rejected

inadequate

discouraged

loss of self control

frustrated

envious

16

" . . . I hear you"

Respond to each of the statements below. On the blank lines, finish the phrase "I HEAR YOU ... "
showing that you have been listening with your heart and really "hearing" what the person is feeling.

Begin each response by "reflecting" what the person is feeling.

EXAMPLE:

My father always takes my kid brother to basketball games. Never me!

*I HEAR YOU . . . your father seems to pay a lot of attention to your kid brother and it makes you feel
neglected and unloved.*

Y'know, no matter how hard I study for the test I know I can't pass. I simply don't understand the work.

I HEAR YOU . . . _____

_____

My boyfriend called off our date to go to the movies on Saturday night. It's the third time he has called off
a date with me.

I HEAR YOU . . . _____

_____

A group of my friends are going to go out Saturday to steal a car and hotrod on the Thruway. I don't want
to go, but I don't want to look "chicken".

I HEAR YOU . . . _____

_____

I'm really tired of my mother expecting me to stay home and take care of my little sister and brothers.
I want to get out and hang out with my buddies.

I HEAR YOU . . . _____

_____

Putting yourself in "someone else's shoes" really means understanding how someone else feels, especially in a situation that can be hurtful and embarrassing. We can win and keep many new friends by putting ourselves in "someone else's shoes".

Read each of the following situations and see if you can identify the other person's feelings. Write what you think each person is feeling on the dotted line. Then write inside that person's shoe what you could say or do to help the situation.

Kevin

A new boy, Kevin, comes into your class in the middle of the year. He is from a far away city. How do you think Kevin feels that first day?

Frightened.   Lonely.

How could you make Kevin feel more at ease?

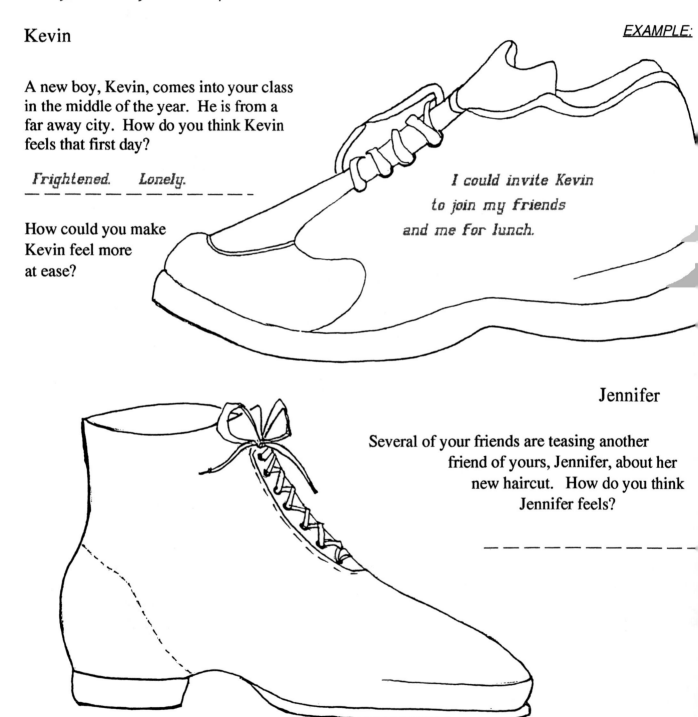

I could invite Kevin to join my friends and me for lunch.

Jennifer

Several of your friends are teasing another friend of yours, Jennifer, about her new haircut. How do you think Jennifer feels?

SOMEONE ELSE'S SHOES

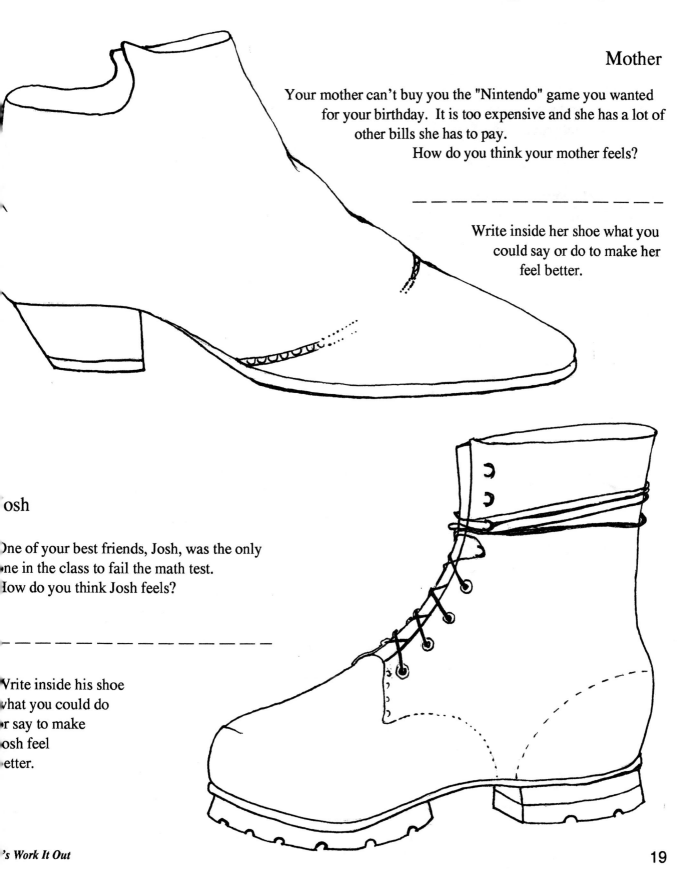

Mother

Your mother can't buy you the "Nintendo" game you wanted for your birthday. It is too expensive and she has a lot of other bills she has to pay.

How do you think your mother feels?

- -

Write inside her shoe what you could say or do to make her feel better.

osh

One of your best friends, Josh, was the only one in the class to fail the math test.

How do you think Josh feels?

- -

Write inside his shoe what you could do or say to make osh feel etter.

Teacher

Your teacher is having trouble getting the class
to quiet down and pay attention.
How do you think your teacher feels?

— — — — — — — — — — — — — —

Write in her shoe what you could
say or do that might ease the
situation.

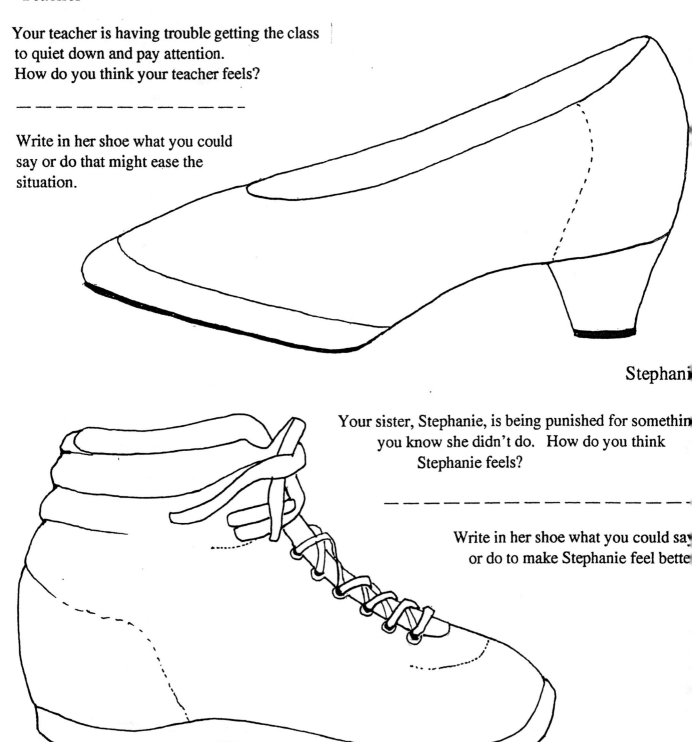

Stephani

Your sister, Stephanie, is being punished for somethin
you know she didn't do. How do you think
Stephanie feels?

— — — — — — — — — — — — — —

Write in her shoe what you could sa
or do to make Stephanie feel bette

SOMEONE ELSE'S SHOES

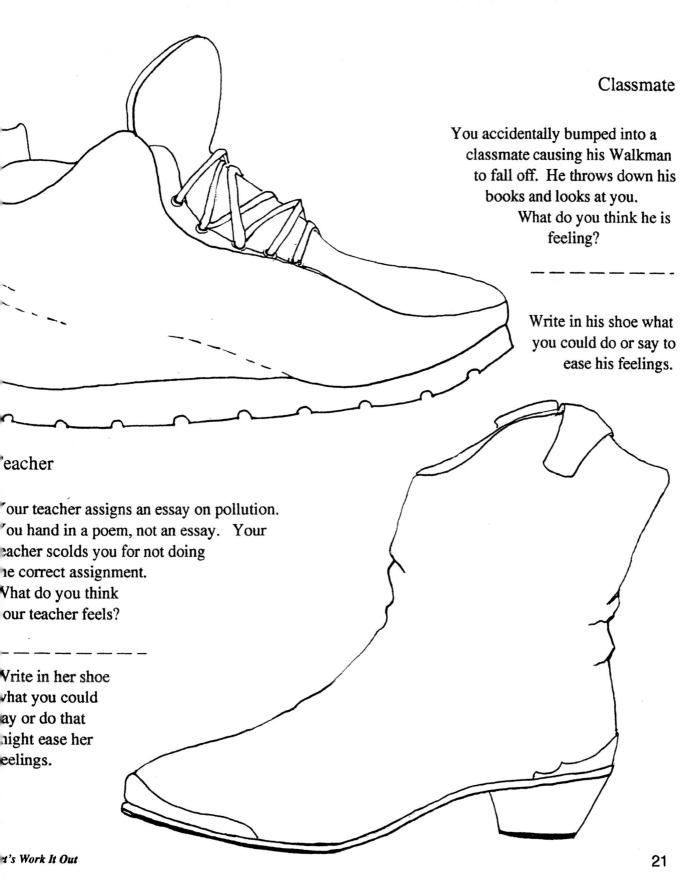

Classmate

You accidentally bumped into a classmate causing his Walkman to fall off. He throws down his books and looks at you.
What do you think he is feeling?

_ _ _ _ _ _ _

Write in his shoe what you could do or say to ease his feelings.

Teacher

Your teacher assigns an essay on pollution. You hand in a poem, not an essay. Your teacher scolds you for not doing the correct assignment.
What do you think your teacher feels?

_ _ _ _ _ _ _

Write in her shoe what you could say or do that might ease her feelings.

BE A MIND READER

After you have read and understood the example below, read what each person is saying in the illustrations on the following pages. Then, write what you think is a thoughtful response in the empty space provided.

EXAMPLE:

La Tasha and her mother have agreed that when she goes out at night, she will return at a certain time. LaTasha goes out one night and returns home after the mutually agreed upon deadline. Her mother has stayed up waiting for her and, when she finally arrives home, her mother yells at her.

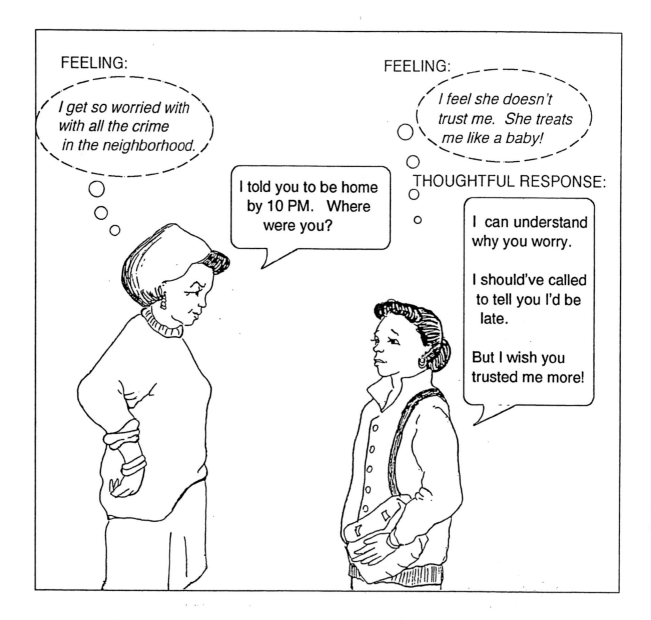

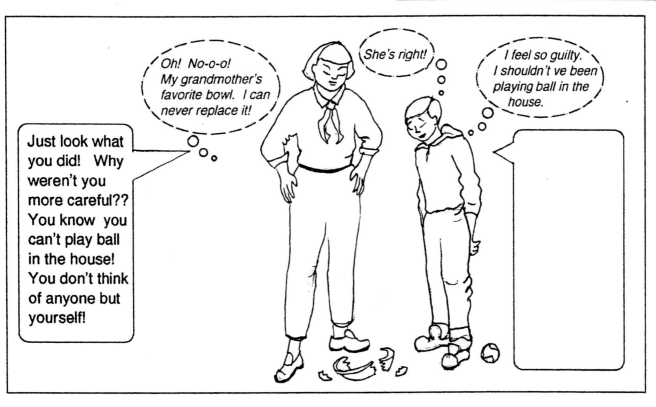

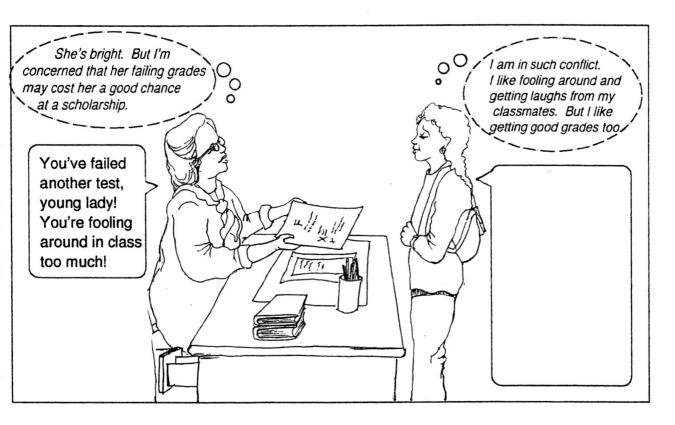

BE A MIND READER

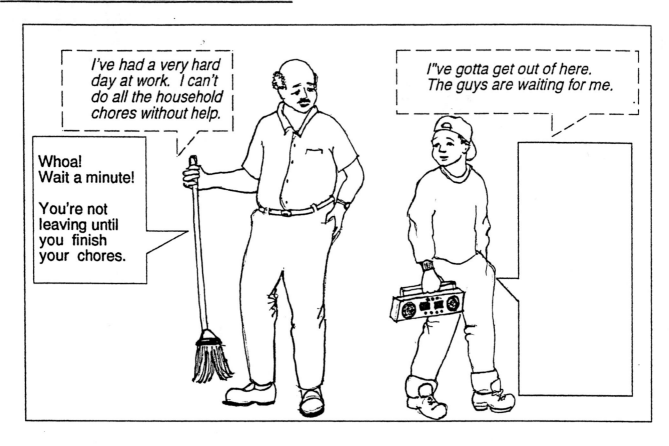

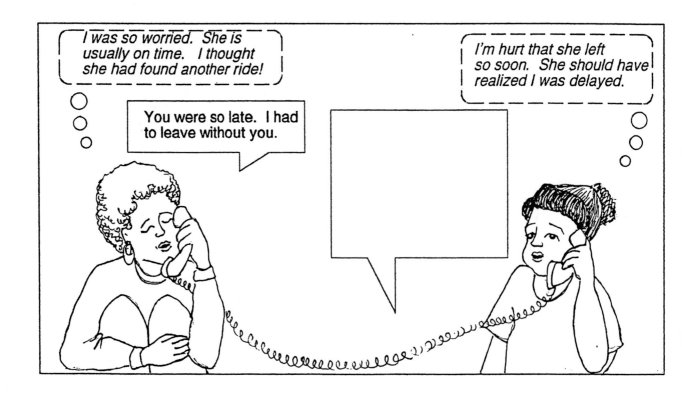

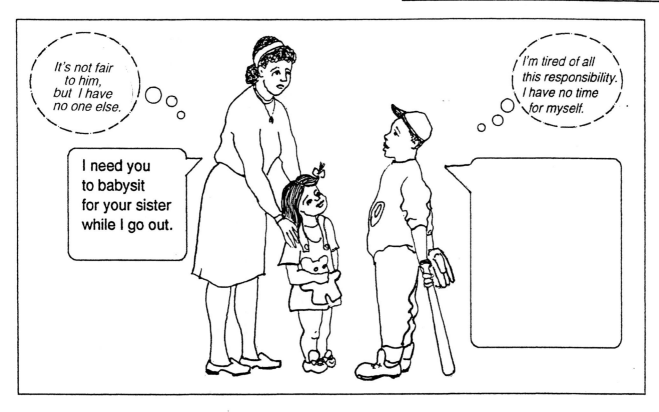

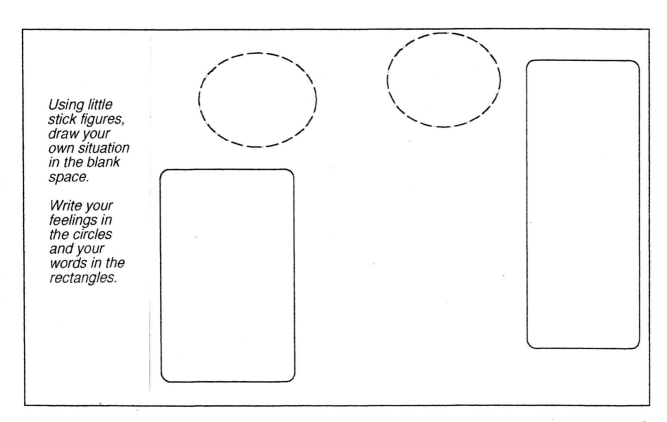

Using little stick figures, draw your own situation in the blank space.

Write your feelings in the circles and your words in the rectangles.

WHY WE ACT THE WAY WE DO

POSSIBLE REASONS FOR BEHAVIOR

TO GET ATTENTION

"Look at me. Notice how noisy and loud (or silly or obnoxious) I am."

I want to be noticed. I need lots of attention. I might not be as smart as others, but I can get attention by being loud or noisy (or silly or obnoxious).

FOR POWER

"I'm the boss. Do what I say."

If I don't boss others around, I feel helpless.

TO FEEL ADEQUATE

"I'm important and can do anything I want."

Unless I act like a "big shot", I feel no one will listen to me.

FOR REVENGE

"I'll get even. Don't mess with me."

I've been hurt. And I'll hurt someone else.

FOR APPROVAL

"I'll do anything you say. Please like me."

I don't feel very likeable for my own self.

Why We Act The Way We Do
Possible Reasons for Behavior

In the following exercise, write some possible reasons for the behavior that is described. Use the examples on the opposite page as your model.

Two students throw coats around the room.

_____

_____

A student sits in the opened window of the classroom and dangles his legs outside.

_____

_____

A student tells all his friends an untrue rumor about a teacher.

_____

_____

A student is very nasty to her grandmother in front of her friends.

_____

_____

A student always volunteers to clean the blackboard.

_____

_____

Some kids always get the latest style haircuts.

_____

_____

Let's Play

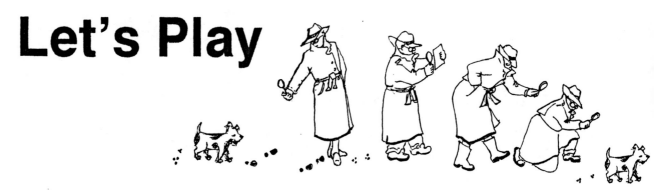

Read each case below. Take your clue from the behavior listed below and offer two or three possible underlying motives, or reasons, for such behavior.

DOING DRUGS

1. _____

2. _____

3. _____

STEALING FROM STORES

1. _____

2. _____

3. _____

HITTING AND SHOVING PEOPLE

1. _____

2. _____

3. _____

BEING A GANG MEMBER

1. _____

2. _____

3. _____

Detective

WEARING A VERY EXPENSIVE
COAT TO SCHOOL

1. _____

2. _____

3. _____

GETTING DRUNK

1. _____

2. _____

3. _____

GETTING PREGNANT

1. _____

2. _____

3. _____

BECOMING TEAM "CAPTAIN"

1. _____

2. _____

3. _____

Now write a descriptive behavior of someone you know and deduce their underlying motive.

_____   _____

_____   _____

what's my personal styl

Circle your responses to the following situations, or write in an additional respo

1. If a friend promised to meet me on a certain corner at a certain time, and she wasn't the I would

> wait fifteen minutes to a half hour
>
> get furious and leave
>
> try to make contact and find out what happened

or, _____

2. If I were waiting on line at the movies and some kids tried to cut in front of me, I would

> let them in line
>
> shove them out of the line
>
> ask why are they cutting in

or, _____

3. If a classmate wrote on my desk, I would

> ignore the whole thing
>
> yell at the classmate
>
> ask my classmate to clean it off

or, _____

Let's Work It

# of problem-solving

4. If a big kid in the neighborhood kept teasing me, I would

> say nothing and try to ignore him/her
>
> tell my parents and family about it
>
> get some of my friends to gang up on him/her

> or, _____

5. If my friend wanted me to steal from a department store, I would

> just go ahead and do it
>
> refuse to and leave
>
> try to dissuade them from doing it

> or, _____

6. If a classmate bullied me every day on the bus to give him/her my home work, I would

> hand it over and keep the peace
>
> tell my teacher and ask for help
>
> ask the bus driver to help

> or, _____

7. If someone took my seat at the movie theater when I went to the bathroom, I would

> find another seat
>
> ask the person to leave or call the manager
>
> curse him/her out and cause a big rumpus

> or, _____

CHILL OUT

This igloo contains may positive ways to control your anger.

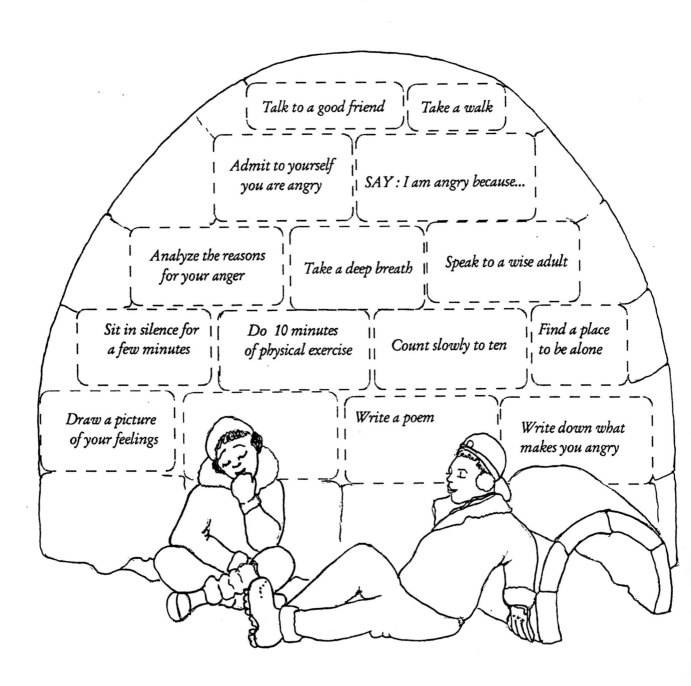

- Talk to a good friend
- Take a walk
- Admit to yourself you are angry
- SAY : I am angry because...
- Analyze the reasons for your anger
- Take a deep breath
- Speak to a wise adult
- Sit in silence for a few minutes
- Do 10 minutes of physical exercise
- Count slowly to ten
- Find a place to be alone
- Draw a picture of your feelings
- Write a poem
- Write down what makes you angry

CHILL OUT

List some things that have made you angry in the past, and why they made you angry.

THINGS THAT MADE ME ANGRY	*WHY THEY MADE ME ANGRY:*

For Example:

Someone borrowed one of my tapes and lost it.

I bought it with my own money and I liked that tape a lot.

1 _____   _____

2 _____   _____

3 _____   _____

Choose one of your examples and describe how you handled or expressed your anger in the past .

_____

_____

_____

Would you handle your anger differently now? If so, describe how you would handle it now. (Look at the ways to control anger in the igloo.)

_____

_____

_____

STAIRWAY to SOLUTIONS

The following is a problem-solving model of the steps you take to reach solutions.

DEFINE THE PROBLEM

1

IDENTIFY POSSIBLE SOLUTIONS

2

EVALUATE SOLUTIONS

3

SELECT A SOLUTION

4

EVALUATE THE OUTCOME

5

efer to the problems described in the
lowing exercise, "Make A Choice".
oose a problem and follow the five steps
the "Stairway to Solutions".

efine the Problem

Identify Possible Solutions

valuate Solutions

elect a Solution

valuate the Outcome

THE TIP OF THE ICEBERG

In the following example, the problem that SHOWS is just the tip of the iceberg. The REAL problem is hidden beneath the surface.

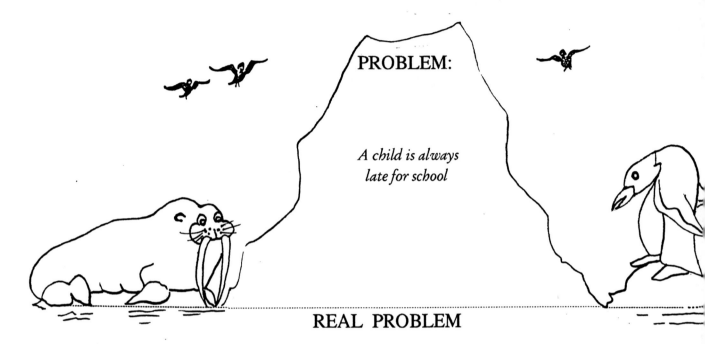

PROBLEM:

A child is always late for school

REAL PROBLEM

Maybe the child wants to stay home in order to get more attention from the mother.

-OR-

Maybe the child didn't do homework and is nervous about getting to school.

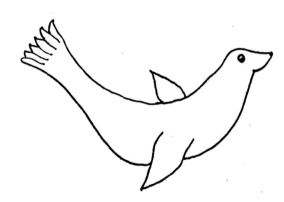

Let's Work

THE TIP OF THE ICEBERG

*What are two of your recurring problems?   Write them in the tips of the icebergs below.
In the hidden part of the iceberg -- below the surface -- write what you think the REAL
problem is.*

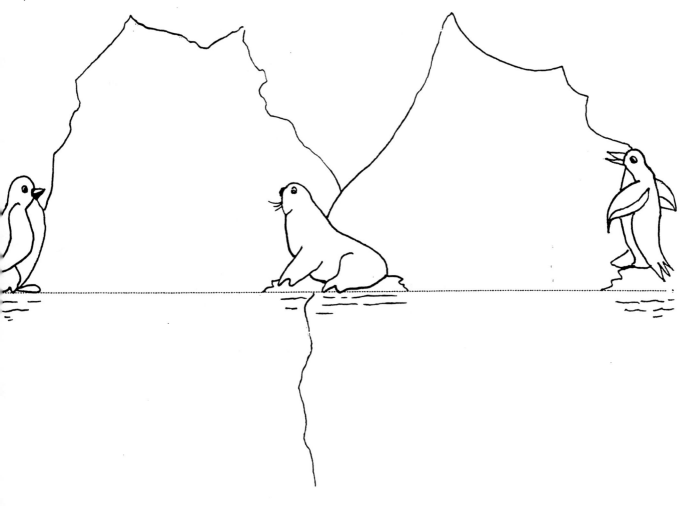

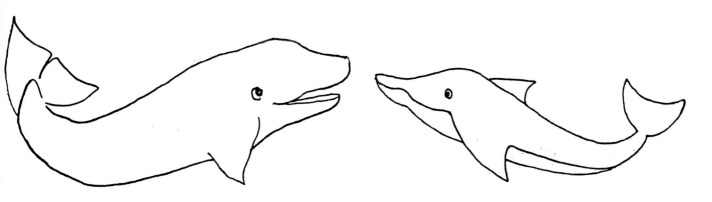

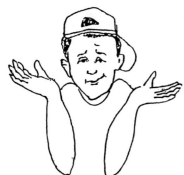

MAKE A CHOICE

Making a choice or taking an action is a lot like throwing a pebble into the water. It causes ripples -- or "consequences". That is why it is important to figure out ahead of time what is the effect of your choice or action.

Below and on the next few pages are situations with choices to make. Read the stories. On the dotted line, write what you think the consequences are for each choice.

1. You are playing in the schoolyard and come across some crack vials on the ground.

    You pick them up and take them home to show your friends.

    ⋯⋯⋯⋯⋯⋯⋯⋯⋯⋯⋯⋯⋯⋯⋯⋯⋯⋯⋯⋯⋯⋯⋯⋯

    You ignore them.

    ⋯⋯⋯⋯⋯⋯⋯⋯⋯⋯⋯⋯⋯⋯⋯⋯⋯⋯⋯⋯⋯⋯⋯⋯

    You tell the teacher what you found and where it is.

    ⋯⋯⋯⋯⋯⋯⋯⋯⋯⋯⋯⋯⋯⋯⋯⋯⋯⋯⋯⋯⋯⋯⋯⋯

    Other Solution and Its Consequence:

    ⋯⋯⋯⋯⋯⋯⋯⋯⋯⋯⋯⋯⋯⋯⋯⋯⋯⋯⋯⋯⋯⋯⋯⋯

2. While throwing something in the garbage, you notice there's a gun in the trash.

    You leave it but tell your friends about it.

    ⋯⋯⋯⋯⋯⋯⋯⋯⋯⋯⋯⋯⋯⋯⋯⋯⋯⋯⋯⋯⋯⋯⋯⋯

    You leave it but call the police to report it.

    ⋯⋯⋯⋯⋯⋯⋯⋯⋯⋯⋯⋯⋯⋯⋯⋯⋯⋯⋯⋯⋯⋯⋯⋯

    You pick it up and open it to see if it is loaded.

    ⋯⋯⋯⋯⋯⋯⋯⋯⋯⋯⋯⋯⋯⋯⋯⋯⋯⋯⋯⋯⋯⋯⋯⋯

    Other Solution and Its Consequence:

    ⋯⋯⋯⋯⋯⋯⋯⋯⋯⋯⋯⋯⋯⋯⋯⋯⋯⋯⋯⋯⋯⋯⋯⋯

MAKE A CHOICE

3. The neighborhood bully, who is known to threaten people with the knife he carries, cuts in front of you at the movie theater.

You shove the bully out of the line and tell him you were there first.

- -

You are angry but you decide it's not worth getting hurt, so you let him in line.

- -

You say nothing but make quiet plans of revenge, real and fantasy.

- -

Other Solution and Its Consequence:

- -

4. Your mother makes you take your little sister with you everywhere you go. She is much younger and cannot do the things you and your friends can. Often this gets in the way of your social life.

When this happens, you throw a fit and scream at your mom.

- -

You yell at your little sister and try to hurt her in a way your mom won't know.

- -

You tell your mom it isn't fair and you walk out.

- -

Other Solution and Its Consequence:

- -

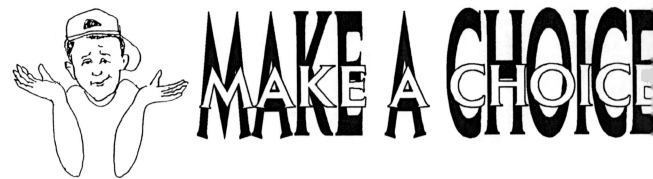

MAKE A CHOICE

5. You break a bowl when you are alone in the house.

   You hide the pieces and hope no one will notice.

   . . . .

   You tell your mother about the bowl and explain that your little sister broke it.

   . . . .

   You admit to playing ball in the house and breaking the bowl.

   . . . .

   Other Solution and Its Consequence:

   . . . .

6. A new girl moves into your neighborhood and many of your friends make fun of her.

   You join in with your friends to tease her.

   . . . .

   You don't join in, but you stay with your friends while they tease her.

   . . . .

   When you are alone, you try to befriend her.

   . . . .

   Other Solution and Its Consequence:

   . . . .

MAKE A CHOICE

7. You have seen someone cheating on a test. The teacher tries to get the class to tell who it was.

> You say nothing.

> -

> You raise your hand and tell the teacher.

> -

> You say nothing but later go up and tell the teacher.

> -

> Other Solution and Its Consequence:

> -

8. While walking home from school you find a can of spray paint. Your buddy suggests using it to write on cars and buildings.

> You go ahead and spray graffiti on a building.

> -

> You throw the can of paint away.

> -

> You give the can of paint to you friend because you're not interested in graffiti.

> -

> Other Solution and Its Consequence:

> -

what's bugging me?

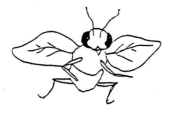 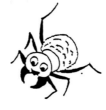 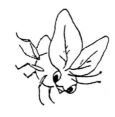 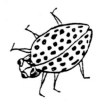

Describe a problem that is always "bugging" you. Use the Stairway to Solutions model on page 34 to help you work it out.

_____

_____

_____

Identify Solutions.

1. _____

2. _____

3. _____

Evaluate The Possible Consequence Of Each Solution :

1. _____

2. _____

3. _____

My Needs Are: _____

_____

_____

_____

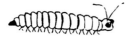 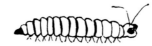

Let's Work It On

what's bugging me?

Other Person's Needs Are:

_____

_____

_____

Choose Your Solution: _____

Steps I Will Take To Reach My Solution:

1. _____   2. _____

3. _____   4. _____

5. _____   6. _____

Evaluate the Outcome: _____

_____

_____

Dear "Problem Solver"...

In the letter below, "All Broken Up" has written to you, the "Problem Solver", to ask for help in solving the problem described in the letter. Please write your answer to "All Broken Up" in the blank "letter" below.

Dear "Problem Saver"

     Last night, I got really mad at my Mom and I broke her favorite vase. I didn't know what to do so I just hid the pieces in my room Now she's asking me if I've seen the vase.

     Should I lie and tell her I haven't seen it and buy her another vase just like it? Or should I tell her the truth? I 'm upset.

                    Yours truly,

                    "All Broken Up"

Dear "All Broken Up"

_____

_____

_____

_____

_____

_____

_____

Your friend,
The Problem Solver

Dear "Problem Solver"...

Write your own letter to the "Problem Solver" describing a problem in your life. Then become the "Problem Solver" and answer it for yourself.

Dear "Problem Solver"

_ _

_ _

_ _

_ _

_ _

_ _

"Don't Know What To Do"

Dear "Don't Know What To Do"

_ _

_ _

_ _

_ _

_ _

_ _

Your friend,

The Problem Solver

Let's Make a Better World

Our universe is made up of many worlds and we are inhabitants of all of them. We live most intimately in our own personal world of school, home, friends and family but, we are also part of the larger world of our neighborhood and town or city. Our country is a member of a still larger world consisting of all nations and all peoples of our planet, Earth.

In this exercise we're going to think of how to make a better world by starting to solve problems in our own smaller world, and then moving on to the problems of the bigger worlds. Don't forget to refer to the five steps of problem solving in the "Stairway to Solutions".

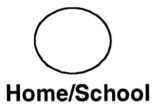

Home/School

Problem:

Possible Solutions:

1.

2.

3.

Let's Make a Better World

Choose two of your possible solutions, and list the steps that need to be taken to achieve the solution.

Steps to Solution # 1

Steps to Solution # 2

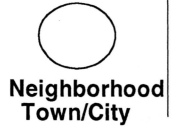

Neighborhood Town/City

Problem:

Possible Solutions:

1.

Let's Make a Better Worl

Possible Solutions: **(Neighborhood/Town/Ci**

2.

.

3.

Choose two of your possible solutions and list the steps that need to be taken to achieve the solution.

Steps to Solution # 1

Steps to Solution # 2

Let's Make a Better World

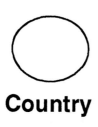

Country

Problem:

Possible Solutions:

1.

2.

Choose one of your possible solutions and list the steps that need to be taken to achieve the solution.

Let's Make a Better Worl

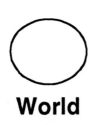

World

Problem:

Possible Solutions:

1.

2.

Choose one of your possible solutions and list the steps that need to be taken to achieve the solutio

Let's Work It

What I Learned About

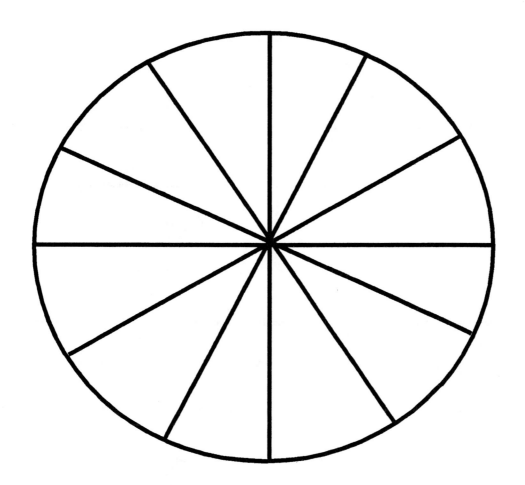

Problem Solving

Fill in the blanks in the wheel with all the things you have learned about problem-solving. The items you list may complete the sentence "What I learned about problem solving is to . . . . . "

building <u>VALUES</u>

achievement	justice	power
wisdom	economic	
religion	loyalty	humanitarian
autonomy	health	pleasure
aesthetic	honesty	recognition

defining <u>VALUES</u>

ACHIEVEMENT --to want to get ahead; to complete all endeavors in the best way possible.

AESTHETIC --to enjoy and appreciate beauty for its own sake.

AUTONOMY --to have control over your own life; to be able to make your own choices.

ECONOMIC --to be wealthy; to have an abundance of material possessions.

HEALTH --to be physically, emotionally and mentally strong.

HONESTY --to be truthful in words, deeds and actions.

HUMANITARIAN --to help other people.

JUSTICE --to be fair to everyone.

LOYALTY --to maintain allegiance to a person, group, institution or other entity.

POWER --to wield influence; to have control and authority over others.

PLEASURE --to have fun; to enjoy all that life has to offer.

RECOGNITION --to feel important; to be given special notice or attention.

RELIGION --to have faith in a higher being.

WISDOM --to know what is true or right and acting or advising in that knowledge.

The VALUE Auction

You are going to participate in an auction of the items listed below. You have an imaginary $2000 to spend any way you want. Before the auction starts, put down the amount you are willing to spend on each item in the "Budget" column. In the last column, put a checkmark down if you won the item.

Items to be Auctioned	Amount You Budgeted	Your Highest Bid	Items You Won
1. To work by yourself without a boss.	$_____	$_____	____
2. A chance to have a money tree growing in your backyard.	$_____	$_____	____
3. To take a nature walk through a beautiful forest.	$_____	$_____	____
4. Earning a trophy in your favorite sport or activity.	$_____	$_____	____
5. A chance to be a helping member of your classroom.	$_____	$_____	____
6. To be the person that people come to for advice.	$_____	$_____	____
7. To have a world without crime.	$_____	$_____	____
A. A chance to choose your own bedtime.	$_____	$_____	____
9. A chance to be the richest person in the world.	$_____	$_____	____
10. To be president of your class.	$_____	$_____	____

(continued on the next page)

The VALUE Auction

Items to be Auctioned	Amount You Budgeted	Your Highest Bid	Items You Won
A chance to redecorate your room.	$_____	$_____	____
An honesty pill so everyone will tell the truth.	$_____	$_____	____
A chance to go to Sunday school.	$_____	$_____	____
A healthy pill that you can take when you don't feel well.	$_____	$_____	____
To be able to settle arguments in a fair way.	$_____	$_____	____
To come to the aid of a friend in need.	$_____	$_____	____
To be a monitor in the schoolyard.	$_____	$_____	____
To always know the right thing to do.	$_____	$_____	____
A chance to improve all your grades on your next report card.	$_____	$_____	____
To be the winner of a Spelling Bee and have your picture in the newspaper.	$_____	$_____	____

(continued on the next page)

The VALUE Auction

Items to be Auctioned	Amount You Budgeted	Your Highest Bid	Items You Won
21. To stick up for your team even when they play badly.	$_____	$_____	____
22.. A world without hate.	$_____	$_____	____
23. To live a long and healthy life for 100 years.	$_____	$_____	____
24. A chance to go away on a religious retreat.	$_____	$_____	____
25. A lifetime supply of computer games.	$_____	$_____	____
26. A chance to be Student-of-the-Month.	$_____	$_____	____
27. A year with nothing else to do but have fun.	$_____	$_____	____
28. To care intensely that everyone gets a fair chance.	$_____	$_____	____

The VALUE Auction

Key to Associated Values in the Auction

1, and 8	Autonomy	10, and 17	Power
2, and 9	Economic	13, and 24	Religion
3, and 11	Aesthetic	14, and 23	Health
4, and 19	Achievement	15, and 28	Justice
5, and 22	Humanitarian	16, and 21	Loyalty
6, and 18	Wisdom	20, and 26	Recognition
7, and 12	Honesty	25, and 27	Pleasure

Choose the three highest items from your Budget and Bid columns in your Auction Values list. Write item numbers down in the columns below. Find the three lowest bids in your Bid column and put those down in the third column.

Then find which value was associated with your item numbers by checking them against the numbers in the Key above. Put the associated value next to its number in the column below. This will help you recognize your personal values.

	Highest Budgeted		**Highest Bids**		**Lowest Bids**	
	No.	Value	No.	Value	No.	Value
FIRST	___	_____	___	_____	___	_____
SECOND	___	_____	___	_____	___	_____
THIRD	___	_____	___	_____	___	_____

DECISIONS . . . DECISIONS

Each of the following sentences describes a situation and offers two choices of action. Circle the one that you would choose. At the end of the exercise read the Key to give you a better understanding of your personal values.

1.   There is a party you want to go to, but you have a test the next day. You choose:

   a. go to the party.   b. study for the test.

2.   You are on your way to the part-time job you have after school and you are going to be late. You notice that an older woman slips and falls to the sidewalk. You choose to:

   a. stop to help the woman.   b. hurry on to the job to be on time.

3.   You notice that a man has dropped $20 out of his wallet at a street fair. You have also been unable to purchase a beautiful bracelet because you were low on money. You pick up the $20 and

   a. return it to the man.   b. buy the bracelet

4.   You have tickets to a ballgame, but your little brother asks you to stay home with him because he's sick. You choose to

   a. give your tickets to a friend   b. go to the game.
      and stay home with your brother.

5.   You find a friend of yours engaged in an argument with a student from another class. They ask you to settle the argument. You choose to

   a. decide in favor of your friend,   b. listen fairly to both sides before deciding.
      no matter what!

6.   You are going to clothing store that is having a big sale. You notice that there are people outside carrying signs accusing the store of paying unfair wages. You choose to

   a. go into the store anyhow and do your   b. decide to shop somewhere else.
      shopping.

DECISIONS . . . DECISIONS

7. A group of friends ask you to hang out with them after school, but you need to go home to work on your part for the school play. You choose

    a. to go home and study your part.   b. to hang out with your friends.

8. You find a carton of cigarettes lying on the sidewalk. Even though you don't smoke because you know it causes cancer, you know you could sell the carton to some of the guys on the corner. After thinking about it you decide to

    a. destroy the carton.   b. sell it to the guys on the corner.

9. You have witnessed a mugging where someone was hurt and are called in to the Police Station to identify the mugger. You recognize that the mugger is a kid who is a bully in your school and you are afraid that he might hurt you if you identify him.

    a. identify the mugger.   b. not identify the mugger.

10. You have designed and sewn an extraordinarily beautiful dress. A local clothing store offers to display it in the window with your name on a placard during the Christmas season. At the same time, a clothing manufacturer has seen it and will buy the design from you for a lot of cash and put it under his own label. You cannot have both deals so you choose

    a. to have your design displayed under your own name in the store window.   b. to accept the cash deal.

Look at the choices you have circled above. Now using this Key, circle the values which have played in your decision-making.

Key to Answers

1.	*a.*	*pleasure*	*4.*	*a.*	*humanitarian*	*8.*	*a.*	*health*
	b.	*achievement*		*b.*	*pleasure*		*b.*	*economic*
2.	*a.*	*humanitarian*	*5.*	*a.*	*loyalty*	*9.*	*a.*	*justice*
	b.	*achievement*		*b.*	*wisdom*		*b.*	*health*
3.	*a.*	*honesty*	*6.*	*a.*	*economic*	*10.*	*a.*	*recognition*
	b.	*aesthetic*		*b.*	*justice*		*b.*	*economic*
			7.	*a.*	*autonomy*			
				b.	*pleasure*			

BAR GRAPH OF VALUES

Count the number of times you have selected a particular value in the "Decisions, Decisions" exercise. Arrange the values in the bar charts below, from the value selected most often to the value selected least often.

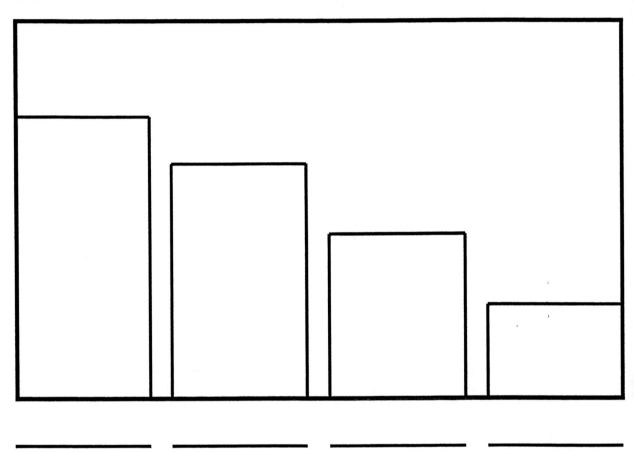

Write the number of times you selected the value in the box and write the name of the value on the line under the box.

Rank order your values from your answers in the Value Auction, page 57, below.

Values and Occupations

Here are some examples of occupations and some of the values associated with them. After reading the list, please answer the questions at the bottom of the page.

OCCUPATION	VALUES
Teacher	Humanitarian, Wisdom
Architect	Aesthetic, Economic
Carpenter	Aesthetic, Autonomy
Health Worker	Health, Humanitarian
Business Owner	Autonomy, Economic
Judge	Justice, Humanitarian

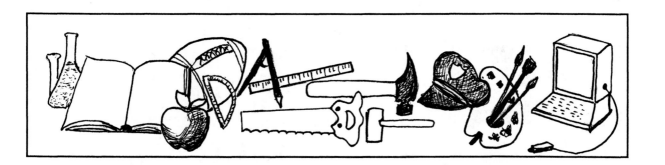

What do *you* want to be when you grow up?

What values are associated with that occupation?

What values do you already have that are associated with that occupation?

What values will you need to develop to do well in that occupation?

PLANET "YOU"

If you were going to start a society on your own newly discovered planet, the Planet "You", what values would you take with you?

Choose the values from the list on page 53 and write them in the Space Ships below.

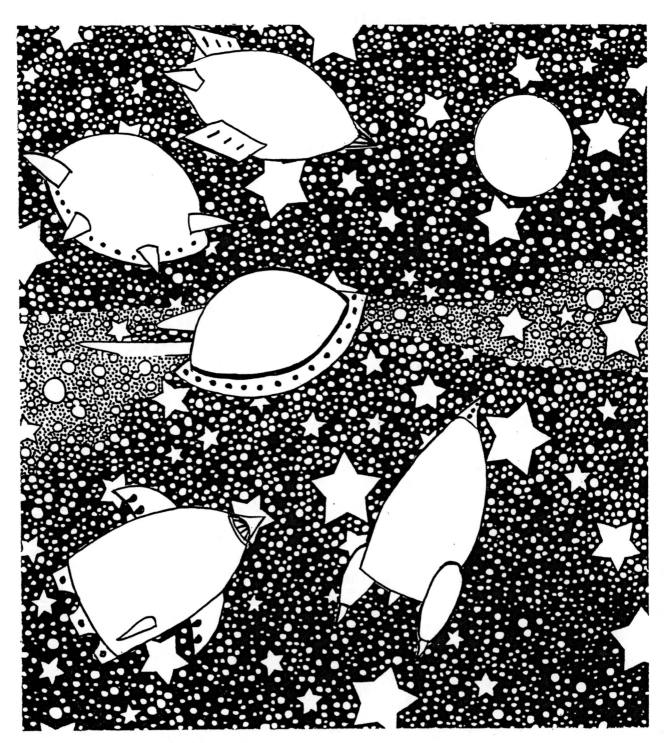

Let's Work It Ou

PLANET "YOU"

Explain how some of the values you chose could make a better world for the people living on Planet "You". Write inside the Space Ships.

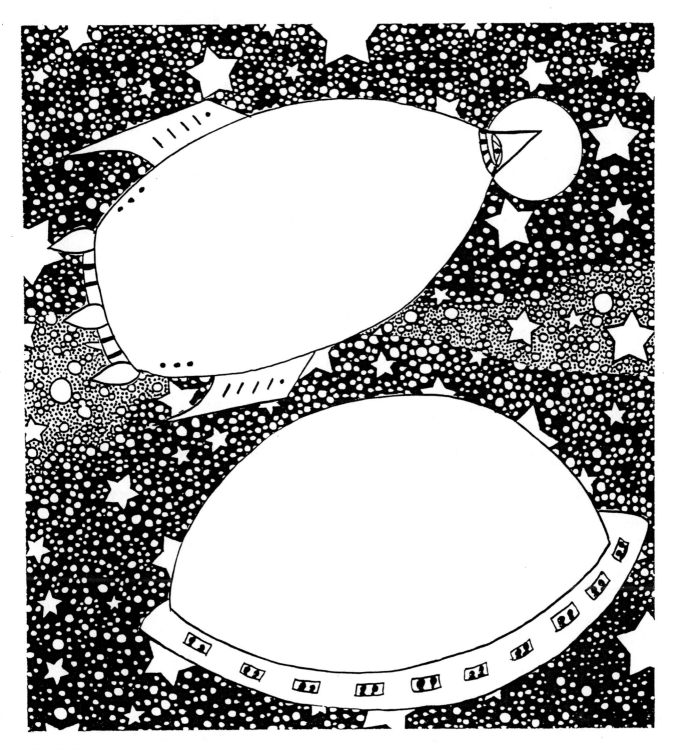

My Problem-Solving Contract

* * I will keep my promises and agreements with myself and others.

* * I will not use "put downs" in my communications with others.

* * I will appreciate what I have and not dwell on what I do not have.

* * I will engage in only positive "self talk".

* * I will correct my mistakes and try to avoid making the same mistakes in the future.

* * I will take responsibility for my own thoughts and feelings, actions and behavior.

* * I will express my thoughts and feelings in positive ways.

* * I will encourage others to express their thoughts and feelings in positive ways.

* * I will try to understand the other person's point of view.

* * I will respect different people's backgrounds: cultural, ethnic and religious.

* * I will not engage in any form of physical or verbal violence.

* * I will respect my health and not use drugs, alcohol or other harmful substances.

* * I will be honest and fair in my dealings with people.

* * I will not abuse power or position against those weaker than me.

* * I will respect persons of the opposite gender, and of older generations.

* * I will work cooperatively for my family, school, neighborhood, country and world.

dated: —————————   signed: ——————————

Let's Work I